MW01232927

The Ultimate Air Fryer Chicken & Turkey Cookbook

Easy Air Fryer Chicken & Turkey
Recipes For Everyone

Alyssa Perry

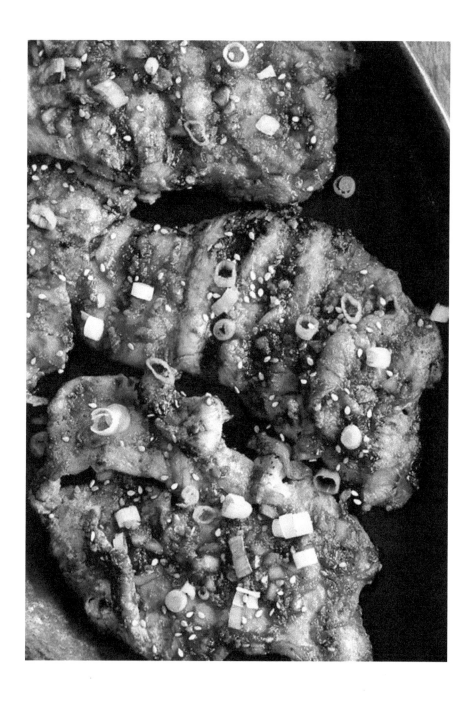

© Copyright 2020 - All rights reserved.

The content contained within this book may not be reproduced, duplicated or transmitted without direct written permission from the author or the publisher.

Under no circumstances will any blame or legal responsibility be held against the publisher, or author, for any damages, reparation, or monetary loss due to the information contained within this book. Either directly or indirectly.

Legal Notice:

This book is copyright protected. This book is only for personal use. You cannot amend, distribute, sell, use, quote or paraphrase any part, or the content within this book, without the consent of the author or publisher.

Disclaimer Notice:

Please note the information contained within this document is for educational and entertainment purposes only. All effort has been executed to present accurate, up to date, and reliable, complete information. No warranties of any kind are declared or implied. Readers acknowledge that the author is not engaging in the rendering of legal, financial, medical or professional advice. The content within this book has been derived from various sources. Please consult a licensed professional before attempting any techniques outlined in this book.

By reading this document, the reader agrees that under no circumstances is the author responsible for any losses, direct or indirect, which are incurred as a result of the use of information contained within this document, including, but not limited to, — errors, omissions, or inaccuracies.

Table of contents

Minty Chicken-Fried Pork Chops

Preparation Time: 10 minutes

Cooking Time: 30 minutes

Servings: 4

Ingredients:

- 4 medium-sized pork chops
- 1 cup of breadcrumbs
- 2 medium-sized eggs
- Pinch of salt and pepper
- ½ tbsp. of mint, either dried and ground; or fresh, rinsed, and finely chopped

Directions:

1. Cover the basket of the Air Fryer with a layer of tin foil, leaving the edges open to allow air to flow through the basket. Preheat the Air Fryer to 350°F. In a mixing bowl, whisk the eggs until fluffy and until the yolks and whites are fully combined, and set

aside. In a separate bowl, mix the breadcrumbs, mint, salt and pepper, and set aside. One by one, dip each raw pork chop into the bowl with dry ingredients, coating all sides; then submerge into the bowl with wet ingredients, then dip again into the dry ingredients. Lay the coated pork chops on the foil covering the Air Fryer basket, in a single flat layer.

2. Set the Air Fryer timer for 15 minutes. After 15 minutes, the Air Fryer will turn off and the pork should be mid-way cooked and the breaded coating starting to brown. Using tongs, turn each piece of steak over to ensure a full all-over fry. Reset the Air Fryer to 320° for 15 minutes. After 15 minutes remove the fried pork chops using tongs and set on a serving plate.

Nutrition:

Calories 262

Fat 17g

Carbs 7g

Protein 32g

Bacon Lovers' Stuffed Chicken

Preparation Time: 10 minutes

Cooking Time: 20 minutes

Servings: 4

Ingredients:

- 4 (5 oz.) boneless, skinless chicken breasts, sliced into ¼ inch thick
- 2 packages Boursin cheese
- 8 slices thin-cut bacon or beef bacon
- Sprig of fresh cilantro, for garnish

Directions:

1. Spray the Air Fryer basket with avocado oil. Preheat the Air Fryer to 400°F. Put one of the chicken breasts on a cutting board. With a sharp knife held parallel to the cutting board, make a 1-inch-wide incision at the top of the breast. Carefully cut into the breast to form a large pocket, leaving a ½-inch border along the

sides and bottom. Repeat with the other 3 chicken breasts. Snip the corner of a large resealable plastic bag to form a ¾-inch hole. Place the Boursin cheese in the bag and pipe the cheese into the pockets in the chicken breasts, dividing the cheese evenly among them. Wrap 2 slices of bacon around each chicken breast and secure the ends with toothpicks.

2. Place the bacon-wrapped chicken in the Air Fryer basket and cook until the bacon is crisp and the chicken's internal temperature reaches 165°F, about 18 to 20 minutes, flipping after 10 minutes. Garnish with a sprig of cilantro before serving, if desired.

Nutrition:

Calories

Fat 17g

Carbs 13g

Protein 36g

Air Fryer Turkey Breast

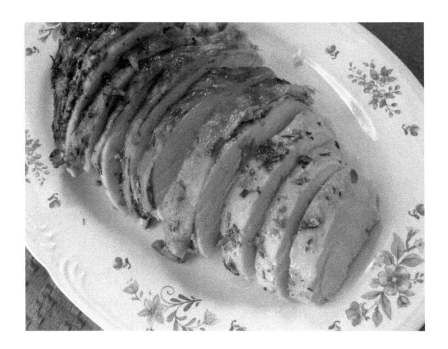

Preparation Time: 5 minutes

Cooking Time: 60 minutes

Servings: 6

Ingredients:

- Pepper and salt

- 1 oven-ready turkey breast
- Turkey seasonings of choice

Directions:

1. Preheat the Air Fryer to 350°F.
2. Season turkey with pepper, salt, and other desired seasonings.
3. Place turkey in Air Fryer basket.
4. Set temperature to 350°F, and set time to 60 minutes. Cook 60 minutes. The meat should be at 165°F when done. Allow to rest 10-15 minutes before slicing. Enjoy.

Nutrition:

Calories 212

Fat 12g

Carbs 6g

Protein24g

Mustard Chicken Tenders

Preparation Time: 5 minutes

Cooking Time: 20 minutes

Servings: 4

Ingredients:

- ½ C. coconut flour
- 1 tbsp. spicy brown mustard
- 2 beaten eggs
- 1 lb. of chicken tenders

Directions:

1. Season tenders with pepper and salt.
2. Place a thin layer of mustard onto tenders and then dredge in flour and dip in egg.
3. Add to the Air Fryer, set temperature to 390°F, and set time to 20 minutes.

Nutrition:

Calories 346

Fat 10g

Carbs 12g

Protein 31g

Chicken Meatballs

Preparation Time: 5 minutes

Cooking Time: 15 minutes

Servings: 2

Ingredients:

- ½ lb. chicken breast
- 1 tbsp. of garlic
- 1 tbsp. of onion
- ½ chicken broth
- 1 tbsp. of oatmeal, whole wheat flour or of your choice

Directions:

1. Place all of the ingredients in a food processor and beat well until well mixed and ground.
2. If you don't have a food processor, ask the butcher to grind it and then add the other ingredients, mixing well.

3. Make balls and place them in the Air Fryer basket.

4. Program the Air Fryer for 15 minutes at 400°F.

5. Half the time shake the basket so that the meatballs loosen and fry evenly.

Nutrition:

Calories 45

Fat 1.57g

Carbs 1.94g

Protein 5.43g

Homemade Breaded Nugget in Doritos

Preparation Time: 10 minutes

Cooking Time: 15 minutes

Servings: 4

Ingredients:

- ½ lb. boneless, skinless chicken breast
- ¼ lb. Doritos snack
- 1 cup of wheat flour
- 1 egg
- Salt, garlic and black pepper to taste.

Directions:

1. Cut the chicken breast in the width direction, 1 to 1.5 cm thick, so that it is already shaped like pips.
2. Season with salt, garlic, black pepper to taste and some other seasonings if desired.
3. You can also season with those seasonings or powdered onion soup.

4. Put the Doritos snack in a food processor or blender and beat until everything is crumbled, but don't beat too much, you don't want flour.

5. Now bread, passing the pieces of chicken breast first in the wheat flour, then in the beaten eggs and finally in the Doritos, without leaving the excess flour, eggs or Doritos.

6. Place the seeds in the Air Fryer basket and program for 15 minutes at 400°F, and half the time they brown evenly.

Nutrition:

Calories 42

Fat 1.44g

Carbs 1.65g

Protein 5.29g

Chicken Breast

Preparation Time: 30 minutes

Cooking Time: 25 minutes

Servings: 6

Ingredients:

- 1 lb. diced clean chicken breast
- ½ lemon
- Smoked paprika to taste
- Black pepper or chili powder, to taste
- Salt to taste

Directions:

1. Flavor the chicken with salt, paprika and pepper and marinate.
2. Store in Air Fryer and turn on for 15 minutes at 350°F.

3. Turn the chicken over and raise the temperature to 200°C, and turn the Air Fryer on for another 5 minutes or until golden.
4. Serve immediately.

Nutrition:

Calories 124

Fat 1.4g

Carbs 0g

Protein 26.1g

Breaded Chicken without Flour

Preparation Time: 10 minutes

Cooking Time: 15 minutes

Servings: 6

Ingredients:

- 1 1/6 oz. of grated parmesan cheese
- 1 unit of egg
- 1 lb. of chicken (breast)
- Salt and black pepper to taste

Directions:

1. Cut the chicken breast into 6 fillets and season with a little salt and pepper.
2. Beat the egg in a bowl.
3. Pass the chicken breast in the egg and then in the grated cheese, sprinkling the fillets.
4. Non-stick and put in the Air Fryer at 400°F for about 30 minutes or until golden brown.

Nutrition:

Calories 114

Fat 5.9g

Carbs 13g

Protein 2.3g

Barbecue with Chorizo and Chicken

Preparation Time: 5 minutes

Cooking Time: 35 minutes

Servings: 4

Ingredients:

- 4 chicken thighs
- 2 Tuscan sausages
- 4 small onions

Directions:

1. Preheat the fryer to 400°F for 5 minutes. Season the meat the same way you would if you were going to use the barbecue.
2. Put in the fryer, lower the temperature to 320°F and set for 30 minutes.
3. After 20 minutes, check if any of the meat has reached the point of your preference. If so, take whichever is ready and return to the fryer with the

others for another 10 minutes, now at 400°F. If not, return them to Air Fryer for the last 10 minutes at 400°F.

Nutrition:

Calories 135

Fat 5g

Carbs 0g

Protein 6g

Roasted Thigh

Preparation Time: 5 minutes

Cooking Time: 30 minutes

Servings: 1

Ingredients:

- 3 chicken thighs and thighs
- 2 red seasonal bags
- 1 clove garlic
- ½ tsp. of salt
- 1 pinch of black pepper

Directions:

1. Season chicken with red season, minced garlic, salt, and pepper. Leave to act for 5-10 minutes to obtain the flavor.
2. Put the chicken in the basket of the Air Fryer and bake at 390°F for 20 minutes.

3. After that time, remove the Air Fryer basket and check the chicken spot. If it is still raw or not golden enough, turn it over and leave it for another 10 minutes at 350°F.
4. After the previous step, your chicken will be ready on the Air Fryer! Serve with doré potatoes and leaf salad.

Nutrition:

Calories 278

Fat 18g

Carbs 0.1g

Protein 31g

Coxinha Fit

Preparation Time: 10 minutes

Cooking Time: 10-15 minutes

Servings: 4

Ingredients:

- ½ lb. seasoned and minced chicken
- 1 cup light cottage cheese
- 1 egg
- Condiments to taste
- Flaxseed or oatmeal

Directions:

1. In a bowl, mix all of the ingredients together except flour.
2. Knead well with your hands and mold into coxinha format.
3. If you prefer you can fill it, add chicken or cheese.
4. Repeat the process until all the dough is gone.

5. Pass the drumsticks in the flour and put them in the fryer.

6. Bake for 10 to 15 minutes at 390°F or until golden.

Nutrition:

Calories 220

Fat 18g

Carbs 40g

Protein 100g

Rolled Turkey Breast

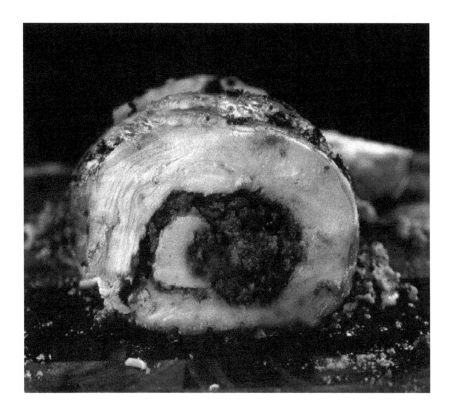

Preparation Time: 5 minutes

Cooking Time: 10 minutes

Servings: 4

Ingredients:

- 1 box of cherry tomatoes
- ¼ lb. turkey blanket

Directions:

1. Wrap the turkey and blanket in the tomatoes, close with the help of toothpicks.
2. Take to Air Fryer for 10 minutes at 390°F.
3. You can increase the filling with ricotta and other preferred light ingredients.

Nutrition:

Calories 172

Fat 2g

Carbs 3g

Protein 34g

Chicken in Beer

Preparation Time: 5 minutes

Cooking Time: 10 minutes

Servings: 4

Ingredients:

- 2 ¼ lbs chicken thigh and thigh
- ½ can of beer
- 4 cloves of garlic
- 1 large onion
- Pepper and salt to taste

Directions:

1. Wash the chicken pieces and, if desired, remove the skin to be healthier.
2. Place on an ovenproof plate.
3. In the blender, beat the other **Ingredients:** beer, onion, garlic, and add salt and pepper, all together.

4. Cover the chicken with this mixture; it has to stay like swimming in the beer.
5. Take to the preheated Air Fryer at 390°F for 45 minutes.
6. It will roast when it has a brown cone on top and the beer has dried a bit.

Nutrition:

Calories 67

Fat 41.94g

Carbs 5.47g

Protein 61.94g

Chicken Fillet

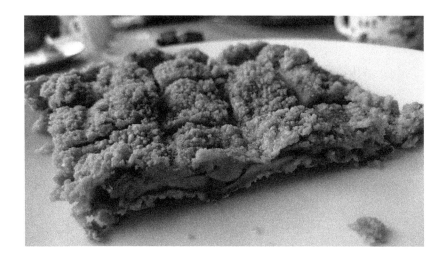

Preparation Time: 5 minutes

Cooking Time: 20 minutes

Servings: 4

Ingredients:

- 4 chicken fillets
- salt to taste
- 1 garlic clove, crushed
- thyme to taste

33

- black pepper to taste

Directions:

1. Add seasoning to fillets, wrapping well for flavor. Heat up the Air Fryer for 5 minutes at 350°F. Place the fillets in the basket, program for 20 minutes at 350°F.
2. With 5 minutes remaining, turn the fillets and raise the temperature to 390°F. Serve!

Nutrition:

Calories 90

Fat 1g, Carbs1g

Protein 17g

Chicken with Lemon and Bahian Seasoning

Preparation Time: 2 hours

Cooking Time: 20 minutes

Servings: 4

Ingredients:

- 5 pieces of chicken to bird;
- 2 garlic cloves, crushed;
- 4 tbsp. of lemon juice;
- 1 coffee spoon of Bahian spices;
- salt and black pepper to taste.

Directions:

1. Place the chicken pieces in a covered bowl and add the spices. Add the lemon juice. Cover the container and let the chicken marinate for 2 hours.
2. Place each piece of chicken in the basket of the Air Fryer, without overlapping the pieces. Set the fryer

for 20 minutes at 390°F. In half the time, brown evenly. Serve!

Nutrition:

Calories 316.2

Fat 15.3g

Carbs 4.9g

Protein 32.8g

Basic BBQ Chicken

Preparation Time: 5 minutes

Cooking Time: 20 minutes

Servings: 4

Ingredients:

- 2 tbsp. Worcestershire Sauce
- 1 tbsp. honey
- ¾ cup ketchup
- 2 tsp.s chipotle chili powder
- 6 chicken drumsticks

Directions:

1. Heat up the Air Fryer to 370°F for 5 minutes.
2. Use a big bowl to mix the Worcestershire sauce, honey, ketchup and chili powder. Whisk it up well.
3. Drop in the drumsticks and turn them so they are all coated with the mixture.

4. Grease the basket of the Air Fryer with nonstick spray and place 3 chicken drumsticks in.
5. Cook for 17 minutes for large drumsticks 15 minutes for smaller ones, flipping when it reaches half the time.
6. Repeat with the other three drumsticks.

Nutrition:

Calories 145

Fat 2.6g

Carbs 4.5g

Protein 13g

Basic No Frills Turkey Breast

Preparation Time: 5 minutes

Cooking Time: 50 minutes

Servings: 4

Ingredients:

- 1 bone in turkey breast (about 8 lb.)
- 2 tbsp. olive oil
- 2 tbsp. sea salt
- 1 tbsp. black pepper

Directions:

1. Warm up the Air Fryer to 360°F for about 8 minutes.
2. Rub the washed turkey breast with the olive oil both on the skin and on the inside of the cavity.
3. Sprinkle on the sea salt and black pepper.
4. Remove the basket from the Air Fryer and spray with butter or olive oil flavored nonstick spray.
5. Put the turkey in with the breast side down.

6. Cook 20 minutes and carefully turn the breast over.

7. Spray with cooking oil and cook another 20 minutes.

8. When done test with thermometer and it should read 165°F. If not, put it back in for a few minutes.

9. Let the breast rest at least 15 minutes before cutting and serving.

Nutrition:

Calories 375

Fat 6.8g

Carbs 8.2g

Protein 15g

Faire-Worthy Turkey Legs

Preparation Time: 5 minutes

Cooking Time: 10 minutes

Servings: 4

Ingredients:

- 1 turkey leg
- 1 tsp. olive oil
- 1 tsp. poultry seasoning
- 1 tsp. garlic powder
- salt and black pepper to taste

Directions:

1. Warm up the Air Fryer to 350°F for about 4 minutes.
2. Coat the leg with the olive oil. Just use your hands and rub it in.
3. In a small bowl, mix the poultry seasoning, garlic powder, salt and pepper. Rub it on the turkey leg.

4. Coat the inside of the Air Fryer basket with nonstick spray and place the turkey leg in.

5. Cook for 27 minutes, turning at 14 minutes. Be sure the leg is done by inserting a meat thermometer in the fleshy part of the leg and it should read 165°F.

Nutrition:

Calories 325

Fat 10g

Carbs 8.3g

Protein 18g

Herb Air Fried Chicken Thighs

Preparation Time: 5 minutes

Cooking Time: 50 minutes

Servings: 4

Ingredients:

- 2 lb. deboned chicken thighs
- 1 tsp. rosemary
- 1 tsp. thyme
- 1 tsp. garlic powder
- 1 large lemon

Directions:

1. Trim fat from thighs and salt and pepper all sides.
2. In a bowl, combine the rosemary, thyme, and garlic powder. Sprinkle over the chicken thighs and press the mixture in putting them on a baking sheet.

3. Cut the lemon and squeeze the juice over all the chicken thighs. Cover with plastic wrap and put in the refrigerator for 30 minutes.
4. Warm up the Air Fryer to 360°F for 6 minutes and spray with butter flavored cooking spray.
5. Place the thighs in the Air Fryer basket, as many will fit in one layer.
6. Cook for 15 minutes, turning after 7 minutes. Check internal temperature to make sure it is at 180°F before serving.

Nutrition:

Calories 534

Fat 27.8g

Carbs 2.5g

Protein 66.2g

Quick & Easy Lemon Pepper Chicken

Preparation Time: 10 minutes

Cooking Time: 30 minutes

Servings: 4

Ingredients:

- 2 chicken breasts, boneless & skinless
- 1 1/2 tsp. granulated garlic
- 1 tbsp. lemon pepper seasoning
- 1 tsp. salt

Directions:

1. Preheat the Air Fryer to 360°F.
2. Season chicken breasts with lemon pepper seasoning, granulated garlic, and salt.
3. Place chicken into the Air Fryer basket and cook for 30 minutes. Turn chicken halfway through.
4. Serve and enjoy.

Nutrition:

Calories 285

Fat 10.9g

Carbs 1.8g

Protein 42.6g

Spicy Jalapeno Hassel back Chicken

Preparation Time: 10 minutes

Cooking Time: 15 minutes

Servings: 2

Ingredients:

- 2 chicken breasts, boneless and skinless
- 1/2 cup cheddar cheese, shredded
- tbsp. pickled jalapenos, chopped
- 2 oz cream cheese, softened
- bacon slices, cooked and crumbled

Directions:

1. Make five to six slits on top of chicken breasts.
2. In a bowl, mix together 1/2 cheddar cheese, pickled jalapenos, cream cheese, and bacon.
3. Stuff cheddar cheese mixture into the slits.
4. Place chicken into the Air Fryer basket and cook at 350°F for 14 minutes.

5. Sprinkle remaining cheese on top of the chicken and air fry for 1 minute more.
6. Serve and enjoy.

Nutrition:

Calories 736

Fat 49g

Carbs 3.7g

Protein 65.5g

Tasty Hassel back Chicken

Preparation Time: 10 minutes

Cooking Time: 18 minutes

Servings: 2

Ingredients:

- 2 chicken breasts, boneless and skinless
- 1/2 cup sauerkraut, squeezed and remove excess liquid
- thin Swiss cheese slices, tear into pieces
- thin deli corned beef slices, tear into pieces
- Salt and Pepper

Directions:

1. Make five slits on top of chicken breasts. Season chicken with pepper and salt.
2. Stuff each slit with beef, sauerkraut, and cheese.
3. Spray chicken with cooking spray and place in the Air Fryer basket.

4. Cook chicken at 350°F for 18 minutes.

5. Serve and enjoy.

Nutrition:

Calories 724

Fat 39.9g

Carbs 3.6g

Protein 83.6g

Western Turkey Breast

Preparation Time: 10 minutes

Cooking Time: 60 minutes

Servings: 8

Ingredients:

- 2 lbs. turkey breast, boneless
- 1 tbsp. olive oil
- 1 1/2 tsp. paprika
- 1 1/2 tsp. garlic powder
- Salt and pepper

Directions:

1. Preheat the Air Fryer to 350°F.
2. In a bowl, mix paprika, garlic powder, pepper, and salt together.
3. Rub oil and spice mixture all over turkey breast.
4. Place turkey breast skin side down in the Air Fryer basket and cook for 25 minutes.

5. Turn turkey breast and cover with foil and cook for 35-45 minutes more or until the internal temperature of the turkey reaches 160°F.
6. Remove turkey breast from the Air Fryer and allow it to cool for 10 minutes.
7. Slice and serve.

Nutrition:

Calories 254

Fat 5.6g

Carbs 10.4g

Protein 38.9g

Lemon Pepper Turkey Breast

Preparation Time: 10 minutes

Cooking Time: 60 minutes

Servings: 6

Ingredients:

- 2 lbs turkey breast, de-boned
- 1 tsp. lemon pepper seasoning
- 1 tbsp. Worcestershire sauce
- tbsp. olive oil
- 1/2 tsp. salt

Directions:

1. Add olive oil, Worcestershire sauce, lemon pepper seasoning, and salt into the zip-lock bag. Add turkey breast to the marinade and coat well and marinate for 1-2 hours.
2. Remove turkey breast from marinade and place it into the Air Fryer basket.

3. Cook at 350°F for 25 minutes. Turn turkey breast and cook for 35 minutes more or until the internal temperature of turkey breast reaches 165°F.
4. Slice and serve.

Nutrition:

Calories 279

Fat 8.4g

Carbs 10.3g

Protein 38.8g

Tender Turkey Legs

Preparation Time: 10 minutes

Cooking Time: 27 minutes

Servings: 4

Ingredients:

- turkey legs
- 1/4 tsp. oregano
- 1/4 tsp. rosemary
- 1 tbsp. butter
- Salt and Pepper

Directions:

1. Season turkey legs with pepper and salt.
2. In a small bowl, mix together butter, oregano, and rosemary.
3. Rub the butter mixture all over turkey legs.
4. Preheat the Air Fryer to 350°F.

5. Place turkey legs into the Air Fryer basket and cook for 27 minutes.
6. Serve and enjoy.

Nutrition:

Calories 182

Fat 9.9g

Carbs 1.9g

Protein 20.2g

Perfect Chicken Breasts

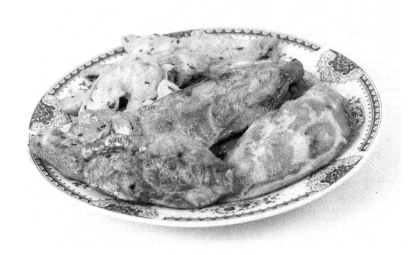

Preparation Time: 10 minutes

Cooking Time: 15 minutes

Servings: 4

Ingredients:

- 1 lb. chicken breasts, skinless and boneless
- 1 tsp. poultry seasoning

- tsp. olive oil
- 1 tsp. salt

Directions:

1. Drizzle oil on the chicken breasts and season with poultry seasoning and salt.
2. Place chicken breasts into the Air Fryer basket and cook at 360°F for 10 minutes. Flip chicken and cook for 5 minutes more.
3. Serve and enjoy.

Nutrition:

Calories 237

Fat 10.8g

Carbs 0.3g

Protein 32.9g

Ranch Garlic Chicken Wings

Preparation Time: 10 minutes

Cooking Time: 25 minutes

Servings: 4

Ingredients:

- 1 lb. chicken wings
- garlic cloves, minced
- 1/4 cup butter, melted
- tbsp. ranch seasoning mix

Directions:

1. Add chicken wings into a zip-lock bag.
2. Mix together butter, garlic, and ranch seasoning and pour over chicken wings. Seal bag shakes well and places in the refrigerator overnight.
3. Place marinated chicken wings into the Air Fryer basket and cook at 360°F for 20 minutes. Shake Air Fryer basket twice.

4. Turn temperature to 390°F and cook chicken wings for 5 minutes more.
5. Serve and enjoy.

Nutrition:

Calories 552

Fat 28.3g

Carbs 1.3g

Protein 66g

Turkey Breasts

Preparation Time: 5 minutes

Cooking Time: 1 hour

Servings: 4

Ingredients:

- 3 lbs. Boneless turkey breast
- ¼ cup Mayonnaise
- 2 tsps. Poultry seasoning
- Salt and pepper to taste
- ½ tsp. Garlic powder

Directions:

1. Preheat the Air Fryer to 360°F. Season the turkey with mayonnaise, seasoning, salt, garlic powder, and black pepper. Cook the turkey in the Air Fryer for 1 hour at 360°F.
2. Turn after every 15 minutes. The turkey is done when it reaches 165°F.

Nutrition:

Calories 558

Fat 18g

Carbs 1g

Protein 98g

BBQ Chicken Breasts

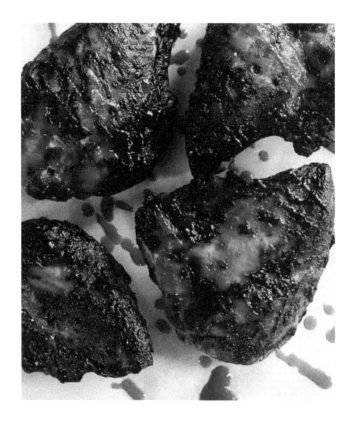

Preparation Time: 5 minutes

Cooking Time: 15 minutes

Servings: 4

Ingredients:

- 4, about 6 oz. each Boneless, skinless chicken breast
- 2 tbsps. BBQ seasoning
- Cooking spray

Directions:

1. Rub the chicken with BBQ seasoning and marinate in the refrigerator for 45 minutes. Preheat the Air Fryer at 400°F. Grease the basket with oil and place the chicken.
2. Then spray oil on top. Cook for 13 to 14 minutes, flipping at the halfway mark. Serve.

Nutrition:

Calories 131

Fat 3g

Carbs 2g

Protein 24g

Rotisserie Chicken

Preparation Time: 5 minutes

Cooking Time: 1 hour

Servings: 4

Ingredients:

- 1 Whole chicken, cleaned and patted dry
- 2 tbsps Olive oiL
- 1 tbsp. Seasoned salt

Directions:

1. Remove the giblet packet from the cavity. Rub the chicken with oil and salt. Place in the Air Fryer basket, breast-side down. Cook at 350°F for 30 minutes.
2. Then flip and cook another 30 minutes. Chicken is done when it reaches 165°F.

Nutrition:

Calories 534

Fat 36g

Carbs 0g

Protein 35g

Honey-Mustard Chicken Breasts

Preparation Time: 5 minutes

Cooking Time: 25 minutes

Servings: 6

Ingredients:

- 6 (6-oz, each) Boneless, skinless chicken breasts
- 2 tbsps. minced Fresh rosemary
- 3 tbsps. honey
- 1 tbsp. dijon mustard
- Salt and pepper to taste

Directions:

1. Combine the mustard, honey, pepper, rosemary and salt in a bowl. Rub the chicken with this mixture.
2. Grease the Air Fryer basket with oil. Air fry the chicken at 350°F for 20 to 24 minutes or until the chicken reaches 165°F. Serve.

Nutrition:

Calories 236

Fat 5g

Carbs 9.8g

Protein 38g

Chicken Parmesan Wings

Preparation Time: 5 minutes

Cooking Time: 15 minutes

Servings: 4

Ingredients:

- Chicken wings – 2 lbs. cut into drumettes, pat dried
- Parmesan – ½ cup, plus 6 tbsps. grated
- 1 tsp. herbs de Provence
- 1 tsp. paprika
- Salt to taste

Directions:

1. Combine the parmesan, herbs, paprika, and salt in a bowl and rub the chicken with this mixture. Preheat the Air Fryer at 350°F.
2. Grease the basket with cooking spray. Cook for 15 minutes. Flip once at the halfway mark. Garnish with parmesan and serve.

Nutrition:

Calories 490

Fat 22g

Carbs 1g

Protein 72g

Air Fryer Chicken

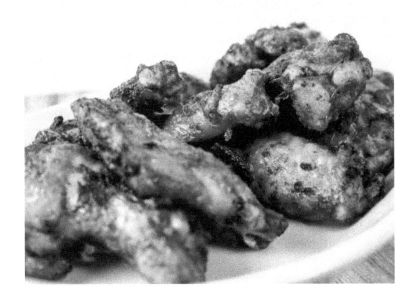

Preparation Time: 5 minutes

Cooking Time: 30 minutes

Servings: 4

Ingredients:

- 2 lbs. chicken wings
- Salt and pepper to taste

- Cooking spray

Directions:

1. Flavor the chicken wings with salt and pepper. Grease the Air Fryer basket with cooking spray. Add chicken wings and cook at 400°F for 35 minutes.
2. Flip 3 times during cooking for even cooking. Serve.

Nutrition:

Calories 277

Fat 8g

Carbs 1g

Protein 50g

Whole Chicken

Preparation Time: 5 minutes

Cooking Time: 40 minutes

Servings: 6

Ingredients:

- Whole chicken – 1 (2 ½ lb.) washed and pat dried
- 2 tbsps. dry rub –
- 1 tsp. salt
- Cooking spray

Directions:

1. Preheat the Air Fryer at 350°F. Rub the dry rub on the chicken. Then rub with salt. Cook it at 350°F for 45 minutes. After 30 minutes, flip the chicken and finish cooking.
2. Chicken is done when it reaches 165°F.

Nutrition:

Calories 412

Fat 28g

Carbs 1g

Protein 35g

Honey Duck Breasts

Preparation Time: 5 minutes

Cooking Time: 25 minutes

Servings: 2

Ingredients:

- Smoked duck breast – 1, halved
- Honey – 1 tsp.
- Tomato paste – 1 tsp.
- Mustard – 1 tbsp.
- Apple vinegar – ½ tsp.

Directions:

1. Mix tomato paste, honey, mustard, and vinegar in a bowl. Whisk well. Add duck breast pieces and coat well. Cook in the Air Fryer at 370°F for 15 minutes.
2. Remove the duck breast from the Air Fryer and add to the honey mixture. Coat again. Cook again at 370°F for 6 minutes. Serve.

Nutrition:

Calories	274
Fat	11g
Carbs	22g

Protein 13g

Creamy Coconut Chicken

Preparation Time: 5 minutes

Cooking Time: 20 minutes

Servings: 4

Ingredients:

- 4 big chicken legs
- Turmeric powder – 5 tsps.
- Ginger – 2 tbsps. grated
- Salt and black pepper to taste
- Coconut cream – 4 tbsps.

Directions:

1. In a bowl, mix salt, pepper, ginger, turmeric, and cream. Whisk. Add chicken pieces, coat and marinate for 2 hours.
2. Transfer chicken to the preheated Air Fryer and cook at 370°F for 25 minutes. Serve.

Nutrition:

Calories 300

Fat 4g

Carbs 22g

Protein 20g

Buffalo Chicken Tenders

Preparation Time: 5 minutes

Cooking Time: 20 minutes

Servings: 4

Ingredients:

- 1 lb. boneless, skinless chicken tenders
- ¼ cup Hot sauce
- Pork rinds – 1 ½ oz., finely ground
- Chili powder – 1 tsp.
- Garlic powder – 1 tsp.

Directions:

1. Put the chicken breasts in a bowl and pour hot sauce over them. Toss to coat. Mix ground pork rinds, chili powder and garlic powder in another bowl.
2. Place each tender in the ground pork rinds, and coat well. With wet hands, press down the pork rinds into the chicken. Place the tender in a single layer into the

Air Fryer basket. Cook at 375°F for 20 minutes. Flip once. Serve.

Nutrition:

Calories 160

Fat 4.4g

Carbs 0.6g

Protein 27.3g

Teriyaki Wings

Preparation Time: 5 minutes

Cooking Time: 20 minutes

Servings: 4

Ingredients:

- Chicken wings – 2 lb.
- Teriyaki sauce – ½ cup
- Minced garlic – 2 tsp.
- Ground ginger - ¼ tsp.
- Baking powder – 2 tsp.

Directions:

1. Except for the baking powder, place all ingredients in a bowl and marinate for 1 hour in the refrigerator. Place wings into the Air Fryer basket and sprinkle with baking powder.

2. Gently rub into wings. Cook at 400°F for 25 minutes. Shake the basket two or three times during cooking. Serve.

Nutrition:

Calories 446

Fat 29.8g

Carbs 3.1g

Protein 41.8g

Lemony Drumsticks

Preparation Time: 5 minutes

Cooking Time: 20 minutes

Servings: 2

Ingredients:

- Baking powder – 2 tsps.
- Garlic powder – ½ tsp.
- Chicken drumsticks – 8
- Salted butter – 4 tbsps. melted
- Lemon pepper seasoning – 1 tbsp.

Directions:

1. Sprinkle garlic powder and baking powder over drumsticks and rub into chicken skin. Place drumsticks into the Air Fryer basket. Cook at 375°F for 25 minutes. Flip the drumsticks once halfway through the Cooking Time.

2. Remove when cooked. Mix seasoning and butter in a bowl. Add drumsticks to the bowl and toss to coat. Serve.

Nutrition:

Calories 532

Carbs 1.2g

Fat 32.3g

Protein 48.3g

Parmesan Chicken Tenders

Preparation Time: 5 minutes

Cooking Time: 10 minutes

Servings: 4

Ingredients:

- 1 lb. chicken tenderloins
- 3 large egg whites
- ½ cup Italian-style bread crumbs
- ¼ cup grated Parmesan cheese

Directions:

1. Spray the Air Fryer basket with olive oil. Trim off any white fat from the chicken tenders. In a bowl, whisk the egg whites until frothy. In a separate small mixing bowl, combine the bread crumbs and Parmesan cheese. Mix well.
2. Dip the chicken tenders into the egg mixture, then into the Parmesan and bread crumbs. Shake off any

excess breading. Place the chicken tenders in the greased Air Fryer basket in a single layer. Generously spray the chicken with olive oil to avoid powdery, uncooked breading.

3. Set the temperature of your Air Fryer to 370°F. Set the timer and bake for 4 minutes. Using tongs, flip the chicken tenders and bake for 4 minutes more. Check that the chicken has reached an internal temperature of 165°F. Add Cooking Time if needed. Once the chicken is fully cooked, plate, serve, and enjoy.

Nutrition:

Calories 210

Fat 4g

Carbs 10g

Protein 33g

Easy Lemon Chicken Thighs

Preparation Time: 5 minutes

Cooking Time: 10 minutes

Servings: 4

Ingredients:

- Salt and black pepper to taste
- 2 tbsp. olive oil
- 2 tbsp. Italian seasoning
- 2 tbsp. freshly squeezed lemon juice
- 1 lemon, sliced

Directions:

1. Place the chicken thighs in a medium mixing bowl and season them with the salt and pepper. Add the olive oil, Italian seasoning, and lemon juice and toss until the chicken thighs are thoroughly coated with oil. Add the sliced lemons. Place the chicken thighs into the Air Fryer basket in a single layer.

2. Set the temperature of your Air Fryer to 350°F. Set the timer and cook for 10 minutes. Using tongs, flip the chicken. Reset the timer and cook for 10 minutes more. Check that the chicken has reached an internal temperature of 165°F. Add Cooking Time if needed. Once the chicken is fully cooked, plate, serve, and enjoy.

Nutrition:

Calories 325

Carbs 1g

Fat 26g

Protein 20g

Air Fryer Grilled Chicken Breasts

Preparation Time: 5 minutes

Cooking Time: 14 minutes

Servings: 4

Ingredients:

- ½ tsp. garlic powder
- salt and black pepper to taste
- 1 tsp. dried parsley
- 2 tbsp. olive oil, divided
- 3 boneless, skinless chicken breasts

Directions:

1. In a small bowl, combine together the garlic powder, salt, pepper, and parsley. Using 1 tbsp. of olive oil and half of the seasoning mix, rub each chicken breast with oil and seasonings. Place the chicken breast in the Air Fryer basket.

2. Set the temperature of your Air Fryer to 370°F. Set the timer and grill for 7 minutes.

3. Using tongs, flip the chicken and brush the remaining olive oil and spices onto the chicken. Reset the timer and grill for 7 minutes more. Check that the chicken has reached an internal temperature of 165°F. Add Cooking Time if needed.

4. When the chicken is cooked, transfer it to a platter and serve.

Nutrition:

Calories 182

Carbs 0g

Fat 9g

Protein 26g

Crispy Air Fryer Butter Chicken

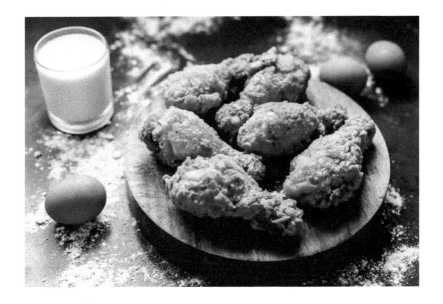

Preparation Time: 5 minutes

Cooking Time: 15 minutes

Servings: 4

Ingredients:

- 2 (8 oz.) boneless, skinless chicken breasts
- 1 sleeve Ritz crackers

- 4 tbsp. (½ stick) cold unsalted butter, cut into 1-tbsp. slices

Directions:

1. Spray the Air Fryer basket with olive oil, or spray an Air Fryer–size baking sheet with olive oil or cooking spray.
2. Dip the chicken breasts in water. Put the crackers in a resealable plastic bag. Using a mallet or your hands, crush the crackers. Place the chicken breasts inside the bag one at a time and coat them with the cracker crumbs.
3. Place the chicken in the greased Air Fryer basket, or on the greased baking sheet set into the Air Fryer basket. Put 1 to 2 dabs of butter onto each piece of chicken.
4. Set the temperature of your Air Fryer to 370°F. Set the timer and bake for 7 minutes.
5. Using tongs, flip the chicken. Spray the chicken generously with olive oil to avoid uncooked breading. Reset the timer and bake for 7 minutes more.
6. Check that the chicken has reached an internal temperature of 165°F. Add Cooking Time if needed.

Using tongs, remove the chicken from the Air Fryer and serve.

Nutrition:

Calories	750
Fat	40g
Carbs	38g

Protein 57g

Light and Airy Breaded Chicken Breasts

Preparation Time: 5 minutes

Cooking Time: 15 minutes

Servings: 2

Ingredients:

- 2 large eggs
- 1cup bread crumbs or panko bread crumbs
- 1 tsp. Italian seasoning
- 4 to 5 tbsp. vegetable oil
- 2 boneless, skinless, chicken breasts

Directions:

1. Preheat the Air Fryer to 370°F. Spray the Air Fryer basket with olive oil or cooking spray. In a small bowl, whisk the eggs until frothy. In a separate small mixing bowl, mix together the bread crumbs, Italian seasoning, and oil. Dip the chicken in the egg mixture, then in the bread crumb mixture. Place the

chicken directly into the greased Air Fryer basket, or on the greased baking sheet set into the basket.

2. Spray the chicken generously and thoroughly with olive oil to avoid powdery, uncooked breading. Set the timer and fry for 7 minutes. Using tongs, flip the chicken and generously spray it with olive oil. Reset the timer and fry for 7 minutes more. Check that the chicken has reached an internal temperature of 165°F. Add Cooking Time if needed. Once the chicken is fully cooked, use tongs to remove it from the Air Fryer and serve.

Nutrition:

Calories 833

Fat 46g

Carbs 40g

Protein 65g

Chicken Fillets, Brie & Ham

Preparation Time: 5 minutes

Cooking Time: 15 minutes

Servings: 4

Ingredients:

- 2 Large Chicken Fillets
- Freshly Ground Black Pepper
- 4 Small Slices of Brie (Or your cheese of choice)
- 1 Tbsp. Freshly Chopped Chives
- 4 Slices Cured Ham

Directions:

1. Slice the fillets into four and make incisions as you would for a hamburger bun. Leave a little "hinge" uncut at the back. Season the inside and pop some brie and chives in there. Close them, and wrap them each in a slice of ham. Brush with oil and pop them into the basket.

2. Heat your fryer to 350°F. Roast the little parcels until they look tasty (15 min)

Nutrition:

Calories 850

Fat 50g

Carbs 43g

Protein 76g

Air Fryer Cornish Hen

Preparation Time: 5 minutes

Cooking Time: 30 minutes

Servings: 2

Ingredients:

- 2 tbsp. Montreal chicken seasoning
- 1 (1½- to 2-lb.) Cornish hen

Directions:

1. Preheat the Air Fryer to 390°F. Rub the seasoning over the chicken, coating it thoroughly.
2. Put the chicken in the basket. Set the timer and roast for 15 minutes.
3. Flip the chicken and cook for another 15 minutes. Check that the chicken has reached an internal temperature of 165°F. Add Cooking Time if needed.

Nutrition:

Calories 520

Fat 36g

Carbs 0g

Protein 45g

Air Fried Turkey Wings

Preparation Time: 5 minutes

Cooking Time: 26 minutes

Servings: 4

Ingredients:

- 2 lb. turkey wings
- 3 tbsp. olive oil or sesame oil
- 3 to 4 tbsp. chicken rub

Directions:

1. Put the turkey wings in a large mixing bowl. Pour the olive oil into the bowl and add the rub. Using your hands, rub the oil mixture over the turkey wings. Place the turkey wings in the Air Fryer basket.
2. Fix the temperature of your Air Fryer to 380°F. Set the timer and roast for 13 minutes.

3. Using tongs, flip the wings. Reset the timer and roast for 13 minutes more. Remove the turkey wings from the Air Fryer, plate, and serve.

Nutrition:

Calories 521

Fat 34g

Carbs 4g

Protein 52g

Chicken-Fried Steak Supreme

Preparation Time: 10 minutes

Cooking Time: 30 minutes

Servings: 8

Ingredients:

- ½ lb. beef-bottom round, sliced into strips
- 1 cup of breadcrumbs
- 2 medium-sized eggs
- Pinch of salt and pepper
- ½ tbsp. of ground thyme

Directions:

1. Cover the basket of the Air Fryer with a layer of tin foil, leaving the edges open to allow air to flow through the basket. Preheat the Air Fryer to 350°F. In a bowl, whisk the eggs until fluffy and until the yolks and whites are fully combined, and set aside. In a separate bowl, mix the breadcrumbs, thyme, salt and

pepper, and set aside. One by one, dip each piece of raw steak into the bowl with dry ingredients, coating all sides; then submerge into the bowl with wet ingredients, then dip again into the dry ingredients. This double coating will ensure an extra crisp air fry. Lay the coated steak pieces on the foil covering the Air Fryer basket, in a single flat layer.

2. Set the Air Fryer timer for 15 minutes. After 15 minutes, the Air Fryer will turn off and the steak should be mid-way cooked and the breaded coating starting to brown. Using tongs, turn each piece of steak over to ensure a full all-over fry. Reset the Air Fryer to 320°F for 15 minutes. After 15 minutes, when the Air Fryer shuts off, remove the fried steak strips using tongs and set on a serving plate. Eat once cool enough to handle and enjoy.

Nutrition:

Calories 421

Fat 26g

Carbs 8g

Protein 46g

Caesar Marinated Grilled Chicken

Preparation Time: 10 minutes

Cooking Time: 25 minutes

Servings: 4

Ingredients:

- ¼ cup crouton
- 1 tsp. lemon zest. Form into ovals, skewer and grill.
- 1/2 cup Parmesan
- 1/4 cup breadcrumbs
- 1-lb. ground chicken
- 2 tbsp. Caesar dressing and more for drizzling
- 2-4 romaine leaves

Directions:

1. In a shallow dish, mix well chicken, 2 tbsp. Caesar dressing, parmesan, and breadcrumbs. Mix well with hands. Form into 1-inch oval patties. Thread chicken pieces in skewers. Place on skewer rack in Air Fryer.

2. For 12 minutes, cook on 360°F. Halfway through Cooking Time, turnover skewers. If needed, cook in batches. Serve on a bed of lettuce and sprinkle with croutons and extra dressing.

Nutrition:

Calories 342

Fat 12g

Carbs 8g

Protein 36g

Cheesy Chicken Tenders

Preparation Time: 10 minutes

Cooking Time: 30 minutes

Servings: 4

Ingredients:

- 1 large white meat chicken breast
- 1 cup of breadcrumbs
- 2 medium-sized eggs
- Pinch of salt and pepper
- 1 tbsp. of grated or powdered parmesan cheese

Directions:

1. Cover the basket of the Air Fryer with a layer of tin foil, leaving the edges open to allow air to flow through the basket. Preheat the Air Fryer to 350°F. In a bowl, whisk the eggs until fluffy and until the yolks and whites are fully combined, and set aside. In a separate bowl, mix the breadcrumbs,

parmesan, salt and pepper, and set aside. One by one, dip each piece of raw chicken into the bowl with dry ingredients, coating all sides; then submerge into the bowl with wet ingredients, then dip again into the dry ingredients. Put the coated chicken pieces on the foil covering the Air Fryer basket, in a single flat layer.

2. Set the Air Fryer timer for 15 minutes. After 15 minutes, the Air Fryer will turn off and the chicken should be mid-way cooked and the breaded coating starting to brown. Flip each piece of chicken over to ensure a full all over fry. Reset the Air Fryer to 320°For another 15 minutes. After 15 minutes, when the Air Fryer shuts off, remove the fried chicken strips using tongs and set on a serving plate. Eat once cool enough to handle, and enjoy.

Nutrition:

Calories 278

Fat 15g

Carbs 7g

Protein 29g

CPSIA information can be obtained
at www.ICGtesting.com
Printed in the USA
LVHW081559160621
690358LV00008B/1137